Basic Wellness Program

A Complete Fitness Diary including Nutrition Guidance and Exercise Plans

- Richa Modak, *M.Sc., M.P.H., RD, ACSM-CPT*

Printed in the United States of America

First Printing, 2020

ISBN: 978-0-578-75665-3

Independently Published

www.richamodak.com

Personal Record

Name:

Address:

Birthdate:

Gender:

Blood Type:

Medications:

Medical Conditions:

Program Start Date:

Emergency Contact:

DISCLAIMER

You should consult your physician or other health care professional before starting this or any other fitness or nutrition program to determine if it is right for your needs. This is particularly true if you (or your family) have a history of high blood pressure or heart disease, or if you have ever experienced chest pain when exercising or have experienced chest pain in the past month when not engaged in physical activity, smoke, have high cholesterol, are obese, or have a bone or joint problem that could be made worse by a change in physical activity. Do not start this fitness and nutrition program if your physician or health care provider advises against it. If you experience faintness, dizziness, pain or shortness of breath at any time while exercising you should stop immediately.

This book (diary) offers health, fitness and nutritional information and is designed for educational purposes only. You should not rely on this information as a substitute for, nor does it replace, professional medical advice, diagnosis, or treatment. If you have any concerns or questions about your health, you should always consult with a physician or other health-care professional. Do not disregard, avoid or delay obtaining medical or health related advice from your health-care professional because of something you may have read in this book. The use of any information provided in this book (diary) is solely at your own risk.

All materials contained within this book (diary) or on our website are for informational purposes only. These materials are not intended to diagnose, treat, cure, and/or prevent any health problems or health conditions – nor are they intended to replace the advice of a physician. You understand and agree that a physician examination and physician consent to proceed with this book (diary) and its contents – "Basic Wellness Program" should be obtained by anyone prior to commencing this program. You understand that this nutrition and exercise program, whether or not requiring the use of exercise equipment and/or other fitness-related activities involve a risk of injury, as well as other health consequences including but not limited to abnormal changes in blood pressure, stroke, other serious disabilities and death, and that you are participating in this program and using equipment and machinery with your own volition and with full knowledge and understanding of all the risks involved. The author of this program, Richa Modak (Rucha Modak), mod-R Nutrition & Fitness LLC and all their staff members and publishers are released, discharged and held harmless from all and any claims, demands, damages or causes of action, present or future, whether anticipated or unanticipated, personal injuries or health consequences, resulting from or arising out of your participation in this program.

In any event, you acknowledge and agree that you assume ALL the risks, injuries and health consequences associated with following the nutrition guidance and exercises / fitness activities with or without the use of exercise equipment enlisted in this program. This program is designed for adults only.

The materials listed in this diary are in no way an alternative to actual medical advice. Please obtain physician consent prior to beginning this program. The directions in this program are based on a general audience. Every person will have different nutrition and exercise needs. Do not consume any foods / drinks that you may be allergic to or have an intolerance to. Please consider any previous and / or current health conditions, diseases and injuries and contact your physician to determine if this program is safe for you.

YOUR USE OF THIS BOOK (DIARY) CONSTITUTES YOUR ACCEPTANCE OF THIS DISCLAIMER.

Dear Reader,

"**CONGRATULATIONS** on taking a step further towards a healthier you! Through this very simple wellness program in the form of a diary, I am hoping to reach out to you and help make it easier to get into a regular fitness routine.

While there are several programs out there, most of them target an established level of exercisers. There are not many resources for those who are looking to strengthen their basics, others who are new to fitness or those who have resumed their fitness journey after a hiatus. Also, the nutrition component, which is key to initiating fat loss, is hardly given due diligence and is very often misleading. So, I have created this easy-to-follow program with a nutrition and exercise diary for you to personalize and incorporate into your routines. This program helps you take small steps at a time so that changes in your nutrition and exercise regimen are gradual and not overwhelming.

As a Registered Dietitian, I have included a simple nutrition guide which explains to you how your meals should be planned in a day and what food categories to consider. This is an important tool for you to design your own meal plans now and in future. When you design your meal plan, ensure that you personalize it based on your schedule, your taste, culture and resources such as availability of local foods. Such a personalized plan becomes easier to follow and adhere to! This program is designed for you to follow at home with basic equipment or at your gym. This diary will serve as your own personal nutritionist and trainer. Results are an outcome of a combination of how motivated you are, whether you stay focused and how well you stay on track. This diary will help you with all of these. Writing down your own goals and recording how you do on a daily basis keeps your mind fully engaged in adhering to the fitness journey you have embarked upon.

This diary makes a perfect resource for you to have at home and it is also a perfect gift – the gift of health! I hope that you enjoy working on this program and pave your way to fitness!"

HOW TO USE THIS DIARY

What is the **goal** of this diary?

This diary is designed for: Adults who wish to work on their basics, those that are new to fitness as well as those who have taken a break from their nutrition and exercise routines and want to restart their fitness regimen. This diary is also very useful to those who have difficulty finding time for exercise due to their busy routines. If used meticulously, this diary will be a stepping stone in changing your lifestyle by helping you take full control of your health.

Often, when we are new to any fitness regimen, we struggle with two important factors: **Time** and **Discipline**. Usually, the reason for failure or giving up is because we set very complicated or unrealistic goals and therefore tend to overwhelm ourselves. The purpose of this diary is to gently introduce or re-introduce you to healthy routines and to help you stay on track. The exercises are designed such that they will not require more than 30 – 45 minutes for completion depending upon how every individual performs the given exercises.

1. Set achievable goals with the guidance provided in this diary.
2. Start with the Basic Wellness Program Level I regardless of your fitness status to set a baseline or to strengthen your basics.
3. Utilize the space provided to enter specifics of your nutrition and exercise, as detailed later.
4. This diary will serve as your "coach" in making the right food choices and in adhering to the food and exercise plans.
5. A series of pictures showing how to perform all exercises correctly is also included. To ensure correct form and posture, we highly encourage you to use this photo guide for exercise instructions.

Following this nutrition and exercise plan and recording all the pertaining details will highlight your strengths. Thus, this diary will serve as a strong motivator, keeping you focused and on track.

HOW TO USE THIS DIARY

This diary is divided into 2 categories:

a. Basic Wellness Program Level I

b. Basic Wellness Program Level II

Each of these levels lasts for a duration of 8 weeks, that is, a total of 16 weeks (4 months)! Accordingly, there are two "food diaries" provided: each one is designed for 8 weeks. Along with this, there are two levels of exercise plans and their corresponding "exercise diaries": each one also designed for 8 weeks.

This particular diary is unique in that it provides you with the tools to create your own, customized nutrition / meal plans. The idea is to follow the meal plans that you create for the entire length of the program, that is for both the levels 1 and 2, while also adhering to the given exercise plan in each level.

The "food diary" is designed for you to record the details of your food intake, with a dedicated space provided to record your water intake.

The "exercise diary" is designed for you to record details of every exercise such as number of repetitions, weights used and any particulars of cardiovascular exercises.

Hence, as you progress and continue to fill out the diary, it will give you an overview of how you have been doing with the program in terms of sticking to both – the nutrition / meal plans as well as the exercise plans.

Additional details on how to fill the respective diary sections is provided later as you read on.

Step 1:

Fill out your current daily routine on the next page. Include details such as –
What time do you usually:
- Wake up
- Eat breakfast
- Go to work
- Come back home
- Eat all other meals in the day
- Cook
- Sleep
- *Etc.*

Based on the routine that you have recorded, establish a suitable time-slot to incorporate your exercise.

My Current Daily Routine

Time	Sunday	Monday	Tuesday	Wednesday	Thursday	Friday	Saturday

Great! Now that you have found a time slot, let us go over some precautions you need to take before you begin...

DO's & DON'T's

What you shouldn't do:

☹ Do NOT push yourself too much

☹ Do NOT continue with exercise if you experience any of the following symptoms, including but not limited to - discomfort, pain, excessive fatigue, shortness of breath, dizziness, bleeding etc.

☹ Do NOT do this program if you have any medical condition or are pregnant, unless advised by your physician

☹ Do NOT ignore previous and / or existing health conditions, injuries, food allergies and intolerances

What you should do:

☺ Contact your physician to determine if this program is safe for you before you start the program

☺ Follow your exercise and nutrition plan

☺ Eat well

☺ Hydrate well

☺ Dress in comfortable clothes while you exercise

☺ Wear good shoes

☺ Maintain good form and posture to avoid injuries

Introduction to the Nutrition Guide

The **Nutrition Guide** in this Diary helps you make your own, customized meal plans through healthy choices. It is very important to create your meal plan because:

Pre-planning your meals lets you focus on choosing and eating a variety of foods. This ensures consuming a well-balanced diet.

For both the exercise levels – Basic Wellness Program Level I and II, we are going to use the same meal plans that you create. How to create these plans and an option of creating up to 5 meal plans is explained in detail in the section "Your Nutrition / Meal Plan".

Hydration is one the most important and often overlooked parameters in fitness. A very simple key on how to ensure adequate hydration is also provided in this section.

During both the levels of this program, you will be recording your food intake and exercise. This way you will be able to monitor:

1. How well could you follow your self-created meal plans?
2. Were you adequately hydrated?
3. Were you regular with your exercise routine?

As you progress, continuing to record these details will serve as a reminder of your strengths and will assist in identifying any deviations from our primary goals of adhering to this exercise and nutrition regimen.

If you happen to miss your exercise someday or consume a meal that is not very healthy, make sure to highlight these instances as you continue to record details. This will help you observe the trend of how you are doing in terms of sticking to your goals; which in turn, will further motivate you to reduce such "highlights" as you progress.

What My RD Recommends:

- Drink Plenty of Water – Check your urine to make sure your water intake is adequate. Refer to the "Pee Key" on the following page.

- Time all your meals evenly through the day.

- Make good food choices instead of following restrictive diets.

- Limit intake of fried foods, processed foods and alcohol.

- Exercise regularly, but never overdo it!

PEE KEY!

Use this Pee Key to ensure that you are hydrated.

Your urine should be light straw colored (numbers 1 and / or 2 in the Pee Key) which means that you are adequately hydrated.

For numbers 3 and above, you will need to increase your water intake.

To ensure drinking adequate water, carry a water bottle with you and make sure that you finish the required amount in a day.

Enter your water intake in your food diary so that you can track your hydration.

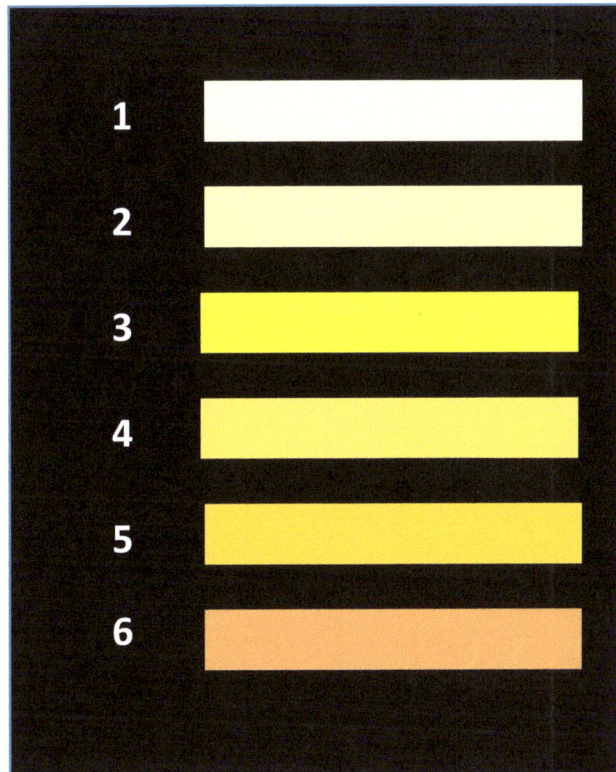

1 – 2: Hydrated
3 – 4: Dehydrated
5 – 6: Extremely Dehydrated

Your Nutrition / Meal Plan

Create your own plan with the guidelines provided on the next pages.

Types of Food

- There are **3** types of macronutrients: **Carbohydrates, Proteins** and **Fats**. They primarily provide us with energy.

- There are **2** types of micronutrients: **Vitamins** and **Minerals**. They help us utilize this energy efficiently and help in normal body functioning.

- All the foods that we consume are further grouped into "food categories" that we need to include in our daily meals.

- Eating a variety of foods from these "food categories" provides us with the macronutrients as well as the essential micronutrients.

These food categories are:

Dairy: Foods from this category are sources of Carbohydrates, Proteins, Fats, Vitamins and Minerals.

Fruits: Foods from this category are sources of Carbohydrates, Vitamins and Minerals.

Vegetables: Foods from this category are sources of Carbohydrates, Vitamins and Minerals.

Whole Grains: Foods from this category are sources of Carbohydrates, Proteins, Vitamins and Minerals.

Lean Meats: Foods from this category are sources of Proteins, Fats, Vitamins and Minerals.

Nuts: Foods from this category are sources of Carbohydrates, Proteins, Fats, Vitamins and Minerals.

Good Fats: Foods from this category are sources of unsaturated fatty acids (Good Fats).

How to Design a Meal Plan

Let us break it down into 3 important categories:

1. Food Variety:

Keep it interesting by choosing a variety of foods at each meal from most or all of the food categories that were listed before. Eating the same foods all the time makes a meal plan boring and subsequently difficult to adhere to! Also, diversity in food choices from the given food categories will provide you with different types of nutrients. To get all types of nutrients from foods, variety in food choices is key! Therefore it is crucial to choose a variety of foods from any given food category.

Example: Let us look at the food category – Fruits. Let us assume that you have planned on including fruits in three of your meals in a day. In that case, instead of including only apples at those three meals, make sure to eat different types of fruits if possible. Such as, apples, grapes and bananas for instance.

There are five pages dedicated towards your meal plans which let you come up with five different options for meal plans. Incorporate all five in your routine so that you avoid consuming the same foods repeatedly. Use your creativity here and enjoy your "self-designed" meal plans!

How to Design a Meal Plan

2. Your Choice: Your choice depends on the following –

<u>Allergies and Medical Conditions</u>: Please consider your allergies and food intolerances before you make a meal plan. Do not consume foods that you may be allergic to or are intolerant of. If you are unsure of your allergies and intolerances, please speak to your physician. Also, consult your physician for any food restrictions that may apply to you due to any medical conditions and diseases.

<u>Taste and Preference</u>: Do not go for foods that you specifically dislike or do not typically eat. For example, if you follow a vegetarian eating pattern, do not plan on consuming meat products. Choose foods that you like and are comfortable with. On the other hand, limit consumption of foods that contain high amounts of saturated fat, trans fat, cholesterol, sugar and salt, even though you may like such foods.

<u>Portion Size</u>: In this program, our focus is on eating a variety of healthy foods and timing our meals. In terms of portion size, your major meals – breakfast, lunch and dinner, should only make you comfortably full. This means that you should not feel sick or uncomfortable as though you have overeaten. Snacks are just for relieving hunger and to provide energy and are not intended to make you full.

How to Design a Meal Plan

3. Meal Timing:

This is one of the crucial aspects of a meal plan. It is important to try and eat your meals at a similar time each day. Each meal should be timed evenly throughout the day. How you time your meals depends on your individual schedules.

In this program our meal plan includes the following meals: Breakfast, Snack, Lunch, Snack, Dinner, Snack, Pre and Post Exercise Snacks. That is a total of 8 meals!

You do NOT have to eat all 8 meals if it makes you uncomfortable. As you progress with your exercise, you may feel hungry. You may incorporate snacks depending on whether you feel hungry later in the program.

If not, you can stick to the basic 5 meals: Breakfast, Lunch, Dinner, Pre and Post Exercise Snacks.

FOOD CATEGORY Examples of foods from these categories are provided on the following page	EATING YOUR MEALS AS DEPICTED BELOW WILL ENSURE CONSUMING A "BALANCED DIET"
Whole Grains	All of your daily meals combined, should contain 50% Vegetables and Fruits. The other 50% should comprise of Proteins (Dairy, Nuts, Beans, Lean Meats), Whole Grains and a small amount of Good Fats [1].
Good Fats	
Dairy	
Lean Meats	
Nuts	
Fruits	
Vegetables	

Food

- Vegetables and Fruits
- Proteins
- Whole Grains
- Good Fats

References:
1. USDA 2015 – 2020 Dietary Guidelines for Americans (https://www.dietaryguidelines.gov/current-dietary-guidelines/2015-2020-dietary-guidelines)

FOOD CATEGORY	EXAMPLES OF DIFFERENT FOODS
Proteins	**Dairy, Lean Meats, Nuts, Beans and Lentils**
Carbohydrates	**Dairy, Fruits, Vegetables, Nuts, Beans and Lentils, Whole Grains**
Good Fats	**Oils – Canola, Olive; Avocado; Nuts etc.**
Dairy	0% or Low Fat Milk, Yogurt, Cottage Cheese, Natural / Processed Cheeses etc.
Lean Meats	Eggs, Skinless Chicken, Skinless Turkey etc.
Nuts	Nuts such as Peanuts, Almonds, Walnuts, Pecans, Pistachios etc.
Whole Grains	Whole Grain – Bread, Tortilla, Roti, Pasta, Cereal etc.
Vegetables	Tomatoes, Cucumbers, Carrots, Celery, Okra, Peppers, Eggplants etc. Leafy greens – Spinach, Lettuce, Kale etc. Lentils, Legumes – Peas, French Beans etc. Beans – Black, Pinto, Garbanzo etc.
Fruits	Apples, Bananas, Berries, Melons, Citrus fruits, Grapes, Cherries etc. Dry Fruits such as Raisins, Cranberries etc.

How to Design a Meal Plan

Let us review what to consider while creating a meal plan:

When you design your meal plans, remember to take into account,

1. Food Variety

2. Allergies & Medical Conditions, Taste & Preference, Portion Size

3. Meal timing

Also remember that 50% or a half of all your daily meals combined, should include fruits and vegetables, both. The other half should comprise of Whole Grains, Proteins such as Dairy, Nuts, Lentils, Legumes, Beans and Lean Meats and a small amount of good fats as depicted in the pie chart earlier.

Remember to combine foods from all or most of the food categories (Whole Grains, Good Fats, Dairy, Lean Meats, Nuts, Fruits and Vegetables) when you design your individual meals. Snacks should be designed only to relieve your hunger and to provide you with energy. Eat smaller portions for snacks. Refer to the earlier tables for guidance, as you design your meal plans.

Design up to 5 different daily meal plans so that you will have plenty of choices. That way, if you run out of groceries for a particular plan, you will always have a back-up plan ready. Also, this will ensure consuming a variety of foods and thus make the meal plans interesting for you to adhere to!

YOUR PLAN Option 1	Now write your own meal plan by combining the food examples provided in the earlier tables. Make sure to include foods from most or all "food categories" per your choice as mentioned before.
Breakfast Time:	
Snack Time:	
Lunch Time:	
Snack Time:	
Dinner Time:	
Snack Time:	
Pre Exercise Time:	
Post Exercise Time:	

PLEASE NOTE!
THIS IS A GENERALIZED NUTRITION PLAN.
DO NOT CONSUME ANY FOODS/ DRINKS THAT YOU MAY BE ALLERGIC TO.

YOUR PLAN Option 2	Now write your own meal plan by combining the food examples provided in the earlier tables. Make sure to include foods from most or all "food categories" per your choice as mentioned before.
Breakfast Time:	
Snack Time:	
Lunch Time:	
Snack Time:	
Dinner Time:	
Snack Time:	
Pre Exercise Time:	
Post Exercise Time:	

PLEASE NOTE!
THIS IS A GENERALIZED NUTRITION PLAN.
DO NOT CONSUME ANY FOODS/ DRINKS THAT YOU MAY BE ALLERGIC TO.

YOUR PLAN Option 3	Now write your own meal plan by combining the food examples provided in the earlier tables. Make sure to include foods from most or all "food categories" per your choice as mentioned before.
Breakfast Time:	
Snack Time:	
Lunch Time:	
Snack Time:	
Dinner Time:	
Snack Time:	
Pre Exercise Time:	
Post Exercise Time:	

PLEASE NOTE!
THIS IS A GENERALIZED NUTRITION PLAN.
DO NOT CONSUME ANY FOODS/ DRINKS THAT YOU MAY BE ALLERGIC TO.

YOUR PLAN Option 4	Now write your own meal plan by combining the food examples provided in the earlier tables. Make sure to include foods from most or all "food categories" per your choice as mentioned before.
Breakfast Time:	
Snack Time:	
Lunch Time:	
Snack Time:	
Dinner Time:	
Snack Time:	
Pre Exercise Time:	
Post Exercise Time:	

PLEASE NOTE!
THIS IS A GENERALIZED NUTRITION PLAN.
DO NOT CONSUME ANY FOODS/ DRINKS THAT YOU MAY BE ALLERGIC TO.

YOUR PLAN Option 5	Now write your own meal plan by combining the food examples provided in the earlier tables. Make sure to include foods from most or all "food categories" per your choice as mentioned before.
Breakfast Time:	
Snack Time:	
Lunch Time:	
Snack Time:	
Dinner Time:	
Snack Time:	
Pre Exercise Time:	
Post Exercise Time:	

PLEASE NOTE!
THIS IS A GENERALIZED NUTRITION PLAN.
DO NOT CONSUME ANY FOODS/ DRINKS THAT YOU MAY BE ALLERGIC TO.

MY MEAL PLAN

I will follow this plan because:

✓ I want to boost up my metabolism.

✓ I want to be healthy and toned.

✓ I do not intend to starve my muscles.

✓ I need energy to focus and concentrate on my work.

✓ I need all these nutrients to remain physically and mentally healthy.

My GOALS for Level I:

I will focus on:

1. Recording my food intake in the Food Diary provided.

2. Highlighting all the meals I think were not healthy.

3. Planning my Groceries ahead.

4. Recording my Exercise in the Exercise Diary provided.

5. Recording my water intake and monitoring my hydration using the "pee-key".

My Personalized Goals for Level I:

How to Fill the Food Diary

Each page is a record for **One Week**.
There are 8 pages for Level 1 and 8 pages for Level 2
corresponding with the two 8 week programs.

Record how much water you consumed.

List all the foods that you have consumed for Breakfast, Lunch, Dinner, Snacks.
Highlight the meals you think were not healthy.

Write the day and date

DAY					
DATE					
BREAKFAST					
LUNCH					
DINNER					
SNACKS					
WATER					
PLAN FOR TOMORROW / GROCERIES					
EXERCISE					
NOTES					

Plan your food for tomorrow and groceries that you will need.

Write in extra details such as snacks, miscellaneous food or beverage intake or medications / supplements etc. in "notes".

Record your exercise as per this plan. (Cardio / Resistance Training / Sun Salutations).

How to Fill the Food Diary

(Sample)

DAY	Monday	Tuesday	Wednesday
DATE	June 1	June 2	June 3
BREAKFAST	Cereal + Oats with 0% milk + fruits +nuts	2 boiled eggs + Whole wheat bread + veggies	Cereal + Oats with 0% milk + fruits +nuts
LUNCH	3 oz. Chicken + vegetable pasta	Egg salad on whole grain toast	2 Wheat Rotis + Lentils + Okra + Cucumber side salad
DINNER	Salad with 1 cup black beans + cottage cheese	Restaurant: Steak + Apple Crumble	3 oz. Chicken + vegetable pasta
SNACKS	10 AM: Apple PreEx - Banana PostEx - chocolate milk	PreEx: Banana PostEx: choc. milk	4 PM: Home made Trail Mix PreEx: Banana PostEx choc. Milk
WATER	2.5 L	3 L	3 L
PLAN FOR TOMORROW/ GROCERIES	Eggs, Spinach, Berries	-	Banana, Almonds
EXERCISE	Arms & Chest	Cardio	Back & Shoulder
NOTES	Extra Snacks: 4 PM - Mango 9 PM - oranges		

How to Fill the Exercise Diary

Write what weights you used. For workouts such as push ups, you may note if you used your knees or did a normal push up.

Write the date

DATE						
EXERCISE	WEIGHT	REPS	WEIGHT	REPS	WEIGHT	REPS
Knee / Std. Push-Ups **Ref: PLATE # 4**						
Shoulder Front Raises **Ref: PLATE # 5**						
Triceps Overhead extensions (Single Arm) **Ref: PLATE # 5**						

Record number of repetitions or reps.

How to Fill the Exercise Diary

Record what exercise you did and all the details that you can fill out. Sometimes, you may not know details such as calories burned or categories such as resistance and incline may not be applicable. In such cases, leave those spaces blank. For the resting week, record how many **Sun Salutations** you did and for how many days with any additional notes.

CARDIO

DAY/ DATE	TYPE OF EXERCISE	RESISTANCE	INCLINE/ OTHER	DURATION	CALORIES BURNT

NOTE:
3 alternate days per week is your Cardio target.
Additional space is provided on these sheets.

RESTING WEEKS

DAY/DATE	TYPE OF EXERCISE	Number	Notes
	Sun Salutations		
	Sun Salutations		
	Sun Salutations		
	Sun Salutations		
	Sun Salutations		
	Sun Salutations		

NOTE:
Resting week occurs after every 3 weeks of the 8 week program. Additional space is provided on these sheets.

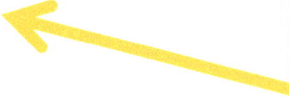

MY FOOD DIARY

This will help me track my food habits. It will also help me monitor how well I can follow my self-created meal plans corresponding with my exercise plans!

Planning my meals and groceries ahead will help me stay focused on my fitness track!

Challenge Accepted! ☺

DAY						
DATE						
BREAKFAST						
LUNCH						
DINNER						
SNACKS						
WATER						
PLAN FOR TOMORROW / GROCERIES						
EXERCISE						
NOTES						

DAY							
DATE							
BREAKFAST							
LUNCH							
DINNER							
SNACKS							
WATER							
PLAN FOR TOMORROW / GROCERIES							
EXERCISE							
NOTES							

DAY						
DATE						
BREAKFAST						
LUNCH						
DINNER						
SNACKS						
WATER						
PLAN FOR TOMORROW / GROCERIES						
EXERCISE						
NOTES						

DAY						
DATE						
BREAKFAST						
LUNCH						
DINNER						
SNACKS						
WATER						
PLAN FOR TOMORROW / GROCERIES						
EXERCISE						
NOTES						

DAY						
DATE						
BREAKFAST						
LUNCH						
DINNER						
SNACKS						
WATER						
PLAN FOR TOMORROW / GROCERIES						
EXERCISE						
NOTES						

DAY						
DATE						
BREAKFAST						
LUNCH						
DINNER						
SNACKS						
WATER						
PLAN FOR TOMORROW / GROCERIES						
EXERCISE						
NOTES						

DAY							
DATE							
BREAKFAST							
LUNCH							
DINNER							
SNACKS							
WATER							
PLAN FOR TOMORROW / GROCERIES							
EXERCISE							
NOTES							

DAY							
DATE							
BREAKFAST							
LUNCH							
DINNER							
SNACKS							
WATER							
PLAN FOR TOMORROW / GROCERIES							
EXERCISE							
NOTES							

WELCOME TO LEVEL-1 EXERCISES

Basic Wellness Program: Level I

Let us begin with the Basic Wellness Program Level I: Exercise Plan.

IMPORTANT: Do not skip any level of this program.

Warm up and Cool down moves are also provided in this guide. Please add your own moves to ensure that you are thoroughly warmed up before you start exercising and thoroughly cooled down after completion of exercises.

Level I GOAL: Work out for 6 days a week for a total of 8 weeks.

In this level, you will perform "Whole Body" Resistance Training Exercises for 3 days per week. Make sure that you do not choose back to back days for resistance training.

For example, if you do your resistance training Day 1 on Monday, then resistance training Day 2 should not be on Tuesday, it could be done on Wednesday followed by Day 3 on Friday of the same week.

For the remainder 3 days of the week, choose any activities from the following:

Cycling / Jogging (outside or on the Treadmill) / Swimming / Elliptical / Walking

Week #4 and #8 are "Resting Weeks" in which you will do only Sun Salutations.

Remember to do your warm ups before any exercise and cool downs after completion of your exercises.

Sample Schedule for Level 1:

	MON	TUE	WED	THURS	FRI	SAT	SUN
Week 1	Whole Body	Cardio	Whole Body	Cardio	Whole Body	Cardio	Rest
Week 2	Whole Body	Cardio	Whole Body	Cardio	Whole Body	Cardio	Rest
Week 3	Whole Body	Cardio	Whole Body	Cardio	Whole Body	Cardio	Rest
Week 4	Sun Saluta-tions	Sun Saluta-tions	Rest	Sun Saluta-tions	Sun Saluta-tions	Rest	Rest
Week 5	Whole Body	Cardio	Whole Body	Cardio	Whole Body	Cardio	Rest
Week 6	Whole Body	Cardio	Whole Body	Cardio	Whole Body	Cardio	Rest
Week 7	Whole Body	Cardio	Whole Body	Cardio	Whole Body	Cardio	Rest
Week 8	Sun Saluta-tions	Sun Saluta-tions	Sun Saluta-tions	Rest	Sun Saluta-tions	Sun Saluta-tions	Rest

The following tables will guide you through your 8 weeks of Level 1. Record your exercise details.

Remember: Week #4 and #8 are "Resting Weeks" in which you will do only Sun Salutations.

For resources on how to perform Sun Salutations, visit: richamodak.com/videos

MY EXERCISE PLAN: LEVEL 1

3 weeks	1 week	3 weeks	1 week
3 days Resistance Training with alternate 3 days Cardio = 6 days/week + 1 day rest	Resting Week! No Resistance Training or Cardio.

Only do **10 – 12** *Sun Salutations* for 4 to 6 days of the resting week. | 3 days Resistance Training with alternate 3 days Cardio = 6 days/week + 1 day rest | Resting Week! No Resistance Training or Cardio.

Only do **12 – 15** *Sun Salutations* for 4 to 6 days of the resting week. |
| | Women: If you have a heavy menstrual flow, try to work around it such that the resting week is also the menstrual week. You may skip the resting week exercises for 3-5 days depending on your cycle. | | Women: If you have a heavy menstrual flow, try to work around it such that the resting week is also the menstrual week. You may skip the resting week exercises for 3-5 days depending on your cycle. |
| **DETAILS OF HOW TO GO ABOUT WITH THE PROGRAM ARE ON THE NEXT PAGE.** | | | |

MY EXERCISE PLAN DETAILS: LEVEL 1

		Weeks 1, 2, 3 GOALS	Weeks 5, 6, 7 GOALS
IN EACH WEEK: Any 3 alternate days: Resistance Training Example: Monday, Wednesday, Friday	**Resistance Training** Whole Body	Focus on Form and Posture; Use lower Weights; lower Repetitions	Increase Repetitions with correct Form and Posture
IN EACH WEEK: 3 remainder days: Cardiovascular Training Example: Tuesday, Thursday, Saturday	**Cardiovascular Training** Choose from: Jogging / Cycling / Elliptical / Swimming / Walking	30 minutes of any Cardiovascular Training	30 minutes of any Cardiovascular Training
Remember: Week # 4 and Week # 8 are Resting Weeks. You only have to do Sun Salutations as mentioned in the earlier table. No Resistance or Cardiovascular Training in these 2 weeks.			

Additional Data (*Body Weight, Body Composition, Waist Circumference etc.*)

WARM - UP BEFORE EXERCISE
Refer to plate # 1 and 2

WARM-UP EXERCISES	REPS	DURATION
Slow Jog on Treadmill / Slow Jog on the Floor in Place / Elliptical / Cycle		5 minutes
Walk / Slow Jog in One Place		5 minutes
Neck Stretch – 2 way **Ref: PLATE # 1**	8-10 each	
Arm Circles (Forward and Back) **Ref: PLATE # 1**	20 each	
Flat Back Hamstrings Stretch **Ref: PLATE # 2**		15-20 seconds
Quadriceps Stretch **Ref: PLATE # 2**		20 seconds each
Foot Roll (Roll your foot at your ankle) **Ref: PLATE # 2**	Both ankles	10 count each

COOL DOWN AFTER EXERCISE
Refer to plate # 3

COOL DOWN EXERCISES	REPS	DURATION
Slow Jog in place	Very Slow pace	About 1 minute
Bend forward, soft knees, relax	Slow and use gravity	15 – 20 seconds
Cat Stretch **Ref: PLATE # 3**	3 - 5	Heart rate should be lower by now
Child's Pose **Ref: PLATE # 3**	–	15 – 20 seconds

MY EXERCISE DIARY: LEVEL I

This will help me track my progress so that I can aim for higher levels of exercise!

WHOLE BODY WEEK 1

DATE						
EXERCISE	WEIGHT	REPS	WEIGHT	REPS	WEIGHT	REPS
Knee / Std. Push-Ups **Ref: PLATE # 4**						
Shoulder Front Raises **Ref: PLATE # 5**						
Triceps Overhead extensions (Single Arm) **Ref: PLATE # 5**						
Knee-bend Lunges **Ref: PLATE # 6**						
One Arm Dumbbell Rows on bench **Ref: PLATE # 6**						
Std. Bicep Curls **Ref: PLATE # 7**						
Std. Crunches **Ref: PLATE # 7**						
Reverse Crunches **Ref: PLATE # 7**						

WHOLE BODY WEEK 2

DATE						
EXERCISE	WEIGHT	REPS	WEIGHT	REPS	WEIGHT	REPS
Knee / Std. Push-Ups **Ref: PLATE # 4**						
Shoulder Front Raises **Ref: PLATE # 5**						
Triceps Overhead extensions (Single Arm) **Ref: PLATE # 5**						
Knee-bend Lunges **Ref: PLATE # 6**						
One Arm Dumbbell Rows on bench **Ref: PLATE # 6**						
Std. Bicep Curls **Ref: PLATE # 7**						
Std. Crunches **Ref: PLATE # 7**						
Reverse Crunches **Ref: PLATE # 7**						

WHOLE BODY WEEK 3

DATE						
EXERCISE	WEIGHT	REPS	WEIGHT	REPS	WEIGHT	REPS
Knee / Std. Push-Ups **Ref: PLATE # 4**						
Shoulder Front Raises **Ref: PLATE # 5**						
Triceps Overhead extensions (Single Arm) **Ref: PLATE # 5**						
Knee-bend Lunges **Ref: PLATE # 6**						
One Arm Dumbbell Rows on bench **Ref: PLATE # 6**						
Std. Bicep Curls **Ref: PLATE # 7**						
Std. Crunches **Ref: PLATE # 7**						
Reverse Crunches **Ref: PLATE # 7**						

CARDIO

DAY / DATE	TYPE OF EXERCISE	RESISTANCE	INCLINE / OTHER	DURATION	CALORIES BURNT

RESTING WEEK

DAY/DATE	TYPE OF EXERCISE	Number	Notes
	Sun Salutations		
	Sun Salutations		
	Sun Salutations		
	Sun Salutations		
	Sun Salutations		
	Sun Salutations		
	Sun Salutations		
	Sun Salutations		
	Sun Salutations		
	Sun Salutations		
	Sun Salutations		
	Sun Salutations		

WHOLE BODY WEEK 5

DATE						
EXERCISE	WEIGHT	REPS	WEIGHT	REPS	WEIGHT	REPS
Knee / Std. Push-Ups **Ref: PLATE # 4**						
Shoulder Front Raises **Ref: PLATE # 5**						
Triceps Overhead extensions (Single Arm) **Ref: PLATE # 5**						
Knee-bend Lunges **Ref: PLATE # 6**						
One Arm Dumbbell Rows on bench **Ref: PLATE # 6**						
Std. Bicep Curls **Ref: PLATE # 7**						
Std. Crunches **Ref: PLATE # 7**						
Reverse Crunches **Ref: PLATE # 7**						

WHOLE BODY WEEK 6

DATE						
EXERCISE	WEIGHT	REPS	WEIGHT	REPS	WEIGHT	REPS
Knee / Std. Push-Ups **Ref: PLATE # 4**						
Shoulder Front Raises **Ref: PLATE # 5**						
Triceps Overhead extensions (Single Arm) **Ref: PLATE # 5**						
Knee-bend Lunges **Ref: PLATE # 6**						
One Arm Dumbbell Rows on bench **Ref: PLATE # 6**						
Std. Bicep Curls **Ref: PLATE # 7**						
Std. Crunches **Ref: PLATE # 7**						
Reverse Crunches **Ref: PLATE # 7**						

WHOLE BODY WEEK 7

DATE						
EXERCISE	WEIGHT	REPS	WEIGHT	REPS	WEIGHT	REPS
Knee / Std. Push-Ups **Ref: PLATE # 4**						
Shoulder Front Raises **Ref: PLATE # 5**						
Triceps Overhead extensions (Single Arm) **Ref: PLATE # 5**						
Knee-bend Lunges **Ref: PLATE # 6**						
One Arm Dumbbell Rows on bench **Ref: PLATE # 6**						
Std. Bicep Curls **Ref: PLATE # 7**						
Std. Crunches **Ref: PLATE # 7**						
Reverse Crunches **Ref: PLATE # 7**						

CARDIO

DAY / DATE	TYPE OF EXERCISE	RESISTANCE	INCLINE / OTHER	DURATION	CALORIES BURNT

CARDIO

DAY / DATE	TYPE OF EXERCISE	RESISTANCE	INCLINE / OTHER	DURATION	CALORIES BURNT

RESTING WEEK

DAY/DATE	TYPE OF EXERCISE	Number	Notes
	Sun Salutations		
	Sun Salutations		
	Sun Salutations		
	Sun Salutations		
	Sun Salutations		
	Sun Salutations		
	Sun Salutations		
	Sun Salutations		
	Sun Salutations		
	Sun Salutations		
	Sun Salutations		
	Sun Salutations		

My Notes: *Include areas you need to improve, ease or difficulty while exercising etc. on this page...*

Did I achieve my goals?

Which ones did I not achieve?

Why could I not achieve them?

What were my strengths?

What setbacks did I encounter?

Congratulations on completing Level I!

WELCOME TO
BASIC WELLNESS PROGRAM LEVEL II

In this level,

1. Continue with your nutrition plan.

2. Continue to make healthy choices.

3. Stick to the exercise routine.

4. Rest well.

5. Do Not Give Up! You are doing Great!

My GOALS for Level II:

I will focus on:

1. Continuing to record my food intake in the Food Diary provided and reducing the number of "highlighted" or "not-so-healthy" food choices that I might make.

2. Limiting all deep fried foods, foods prepared with refined flours such as cakes, cookies, white bread etc. to 0-1 times per week.

3. Trying to eat homemade food as much as possible by planning my groceries ahead.

4. Disciplining myself to adhere to my nutrition and exercise plan rigidly.

5. Staying well-hydrated.

My Personalized Goals for Level II:

DAY							
DATE							
BREAKFAST							
LUNCH							
DINNER							
SNACKS							
WATER							
PLAN FOR TOMORROW / GROCERIES							
EXERCISE							
NOTES							

DAY						
DATE						
BREAKFAST						
LUNCH						
DINNER						
SNACKS						
WATER						
PLAN FOR TOMORROW / GROCERIES						
EXERCISE						
NOTES						

DAY						
DATE						
BREAKFAST						
LUNCH						
DINNER						
SNACKS						
WATER						
PLAN FOR TOMORROW / GROCERIES						
EXERCISE						
NOTES						

DAY						
DATE						
BREAKFAST						
LUNCH						
DINNER						
SNACKS						
WATER						
PLAN FOR TOMORROW / GROCERIES						
EXERCISE						
NOTES						

DAY						
DATE						
BREAKFAST						
LUNCH						
DINNER						
SNACKS						
WATER						
PLAN FOR TOMORROW / GROCERIES						
EXERCISE						
NOTES						

DAY						
DATE						
BREAKFAST						
LUNCH						
DINNER						
SNACKS						
WATER						
PLAN FOR TOMORROW / GROCERIES						
EXERCISE						
NOTES						

DAY							
DATE							
BREAKFAST							
LUNCH							
DINNER							
SNACKS							
WATER							
PLAN FOR TOMORROW / GROCERIES							
EXERCISE							
NOTES							

DAY							
DATE							
BREAKFAST							
LUNCH							
DINNER							
SNACKS							
WATER							
PLAN FOR TOMORROW / GROCERIES							
EXERCISE							
NOTES							

WELCOME TO LEVEL-2 EXERCISES

Basic Wellness Program: Level II

Let us now begin with the Basic Wellness Program Level II: Exercise Plan. This level introduces you to isolating different muscle groups and working each muscle group out. Use the same warm up and cool down as before. Remember to add your own moves to ensure that you are thoroughly warmed up before you start exercising and thoroughly cooled down after completion of exercises.

REMEMBER: One day missed is one muscle group missed! Do not skip any days!

Level II GOAL: Work out 6 days a week for a total of 8 weeks.

In this level, you do your resistance training for 3 days per week. Make sure that you do not choose back to back days for resistance training. The muscle groups will be divided as follows:

In each ONE Week:

Day 1: Arms and Chest

Day 2: Cardio

Day 3: Back and Shoulders

Day 4: Cardio

Day 5: Legs and Core

Day 6: Cardio

Day 7: Rest

Sample Schedule for Level 2:

	MON	TUE	WED	THURS	FRI	SAT	SUN
Week 1	Arms & Chest	Cardio	Back & Shoulders	Cardio	Legs & Core	Cardio	Rest
Week 2	Arms & Chest	Cardio	Back & Shoulders	Cardio	Legs & Core	Cardio	Rest
Week 3	Arms & Chest	Cardio	Back & Shoulders	Cardio	Legs & Core	Cardio	Rest
Week 4	Sun Saluta-tions	Sun Saluta-tions	Rest	Sun Saluta-tions	Sun Saluta-tions	Sun Saluta-tions	Rest
Week 5	Arms & Chest	Cardio	Back & Shoulders	Cardio	Legs & Core	Cardio	Rest
Week 6	Arms & Chest	Cardio	Back & Shoulders	Cardio	Legs & Core	Cardio	Rest
Week 7	Arms & Chest	Cardio	Back & Shoulders	Cardio	Legs & Core	Cardio	Rest
Week 8	Sun Saluta-tions	Sun Saluta-tions	Sun Saluta-tions	Sun Saluta-tions	Sun Saluta-tions	Sun Saluta-tions	Rest

The following tables will guide you through your 8 weeks of Level 2. Record your exercise details.

Remember: Week #4 and #8 are "Resting Weeks" in which you will do only Sun Salutations.

For resources on how to perform Sun Salutations, visit: richamodak.com/videos

MY EXERCISE PLAN: LEVEL 2

3 weeks	1 week	3 weeks	1 week
3 days Resistance Training with alternate 3 days Cardio = 6 days/week + 1 day rest	Resting Week! No Resistance Training or Cardio. Only do **10 - 15** ***Sun Salutations*** for 5 to 6 days of the resting week. You may increase this number if you feel comfortable.	3 days Resistance Training with alternate 3 days Cardio = 6 days/week + 1 day rest	Resting Week! No Resistance Training or Cardio. Only do **15 - 20** ***Sun Salutations*** for 5 to 6 days of the resting week. You may increase this number if you feel comfortable.
	Women: If you have a heavy menstrual flow, try to work around it such that the resting week is also the menstrual week. You may skip the resting week exercises for 3-5 days depending on your cycle.		Women: If you have a heavy menstrual flow, try to work around it such that the resting week is also the menstrual week. You may skip the resting week exercises for 3-5 days depending on your cycle.
DETAILS OF HOW TO GO ABOUT WITH THE PROGRAM ARE ON THE NEXT PAGE.			

MY EXERCISE PLAN DETAILS: LEVEL 2

		Weeks 1, 2, 3 GOALS	Weeks 5, 6, 7 GOALS
IN EACH WEEK: Any 3 alternate days: Resistance Training Example: Monday, Wednesday, Friday.	**Resistance Training:** Arms & Chest, Back & Shoulders, Legs & Core	Focus on Form and Posture; Use lower weights; Lower Repetitions	Increase Repetitions with correct Form and Posture; Increase Weights gradually and only if comfortable
IN EACH WEEK: 3 remainder days: Cardiovascular Training Example: Tuesday Thursday Saturday	**Cardiovascular Training** Choose from: Jogging / Cycling / Elliptical / Swimming	45 minutes of any Cardiovascular Training	45 minutes of any Cardiovascular Training
Remember: Week # 4 and Week # 8 are Resting Weeks. You only have to do Sun Salutations as mentioned in the earlier table. No Resistance or Cardiovascular Training in these 2 weeks.			

Additional Data (*Body Weight, Body Composition, Waist Circumference etc.*)

WARM- UP BEFORE EXERCISE
Refer to plate # 1 and 2

WARM-UP EXERCISES	REPS	DURATION
Slow Jog on Treadmill / Slow Jog on the Floor in Place / Elliptical / Cycle		5 minutes
Walk / Slow Jog in One Place		5 minutes
Neck Stretch – 2 way **Ref: PLATE # 1**	8-10 each	
Arm Circles (Forward and Back) **Ref: PLATE # 1**	20 each	
Flat Back Hamstrings Stretch **Ref: PLATE # 2**		15-20 seconds
Quadriceps Stretch **Ref: PLATE # 2**		20 seconds each
Foot Roll (Roll your foot at your ankle) **Ref: PLATE # 2**	Both ankles	10 count each

COOL DOWN AFTER EXERCISE
Refer to plate # 3

COOL DOWN EXERCISES	REPS	DURATION
Slow Jog in place	Very Slow pace	About 1 minute
Bend forward, soft knees, relax	Slow and use gravity	15 – 20 seconds
Cat Stretch **Ref: PLATE # 3**	3 - 5	Heart rate should be lower by now
Child's Pose **Ref: PLATE # 3**	–	15 – 20 seconds

MY EXERCISE DIARY LEVEL II

I'm all set to start Level II.
Let's do this!!!

ARMS & CHEST

EXERCISE	DATE					
	WEIGHT	REPS	WEIGHT	REPS	WEIGHT	REPS
Knee or Std. Push Ups **Ref: PLATE # 4**						
Std. Biceps Curls **Ref: PLATE # 7**						
Triceps Overhead extensions (Single Arm) **Ref: PLATE # 5**						
Knee or Std. Push-Ups **Ref: PLATE # 4**						
Hammer Biceps Curls **Ref: PLATE # 8**						
Triceps Overhead extensions (Single Arm) **Ref: PLATE # 5**						
Knee or Std. Push-Ups **Ref: PLATE # 4**						
Single Arm Biceps Curls **Ref: PLATE # 8**						
Triceps Dips **Ref: PLATE # 9**						

BACK & SHOULDERS

EXERCISE	DATE					
	WEIGHT	REPS	WEIGHT	REPS	WEIGHT	REPS
One Arm Dumbbell Rows on Bench **Ref: PLATE # 6**						
Shoulder Front Raises **Ref: PLATE # 5**						
Std. Pull Ups **Ref: PLATE # 10**						
Shoulder Press **Ref: PLATE # 10**						
Narrow Grip Pull Ups **Ref: PLATE # 11**						
Shoulder Lateral Raises **Ref: PLATE # 9**						
Wide Pull Ups **Ref: PLATE # 11**						
Shoulder Press **Ref: PLATE # 10**						

LEGS & CORE

EXERCISE	DATE					
	WEIGHT	REPS	WEIGHT	REPS	WEIGHT	REPS
Knee Bend Lunges **Ref: PLATE # 6**						
Deep Squats **Ref: PLATE # 12**						
Std. Crunches **Ref: PLATE # 7**						
Straight Back-Leg Lunges **Ref: PLATE # 12**						
Calf Raises **Ref: PLATE # 13**						
Piano Crunches **Ref: PLATE # 13**						
Chair Pose Hold **Ref: PLATE # 14**						
Demi Squats **Ref: PLATE # 14**						
Reverse Crunches **Ref: PLATE # 7**						

CARDIO

DAY / DATE	TYPE OF EXERCISE	RESISTANCE	INCLINE / OTHER	DURATION	CALORIES BURNT

RESTING WEEK

DAY/DATE	TYPE OF EXERCISE	Number	Notes
	Sun Salutations		
	Sun Salutations		
	Sun Salutations		
	Sun Salutations		
	Sun Salutations		
	Sun Salutations		
	Sun Salutations		
	Sun Salutations		
	Sun Salutations		
	Sun Salutations		
	Sun Salutations		
	Sun Salutations		

ARMS & CHEST

EXERCISE	DATE					
	WEIGHT	REPS	WEIGHT	REPS	WEIGHT	REPS
Knee or Std. Push Ups **Ref: PLATE # 4**						
Std. Biceps Curls **Ref: PLATE # 7**						
Triceps Overhead extensions (Single Arm) **Ref: PLATE # 5**						
Knee or Std. Push-Ups **Ref: PLATE # 4**						
Hammer Biceps Curls **Ref: PLATE # 8**						
Triceps Overhead extensions (Single Arm) **Ref: PLATE # 5**						
Knee or Std. Push-Ups **Ref: PLATE # 4**						
Single Arm Biceps Curls **Ref: PLATE # 8**						
Triceps Dips **Ref: PLATE # 9**						

BACK & SHOULDERS

	DATE						
EXERCISE	WEIGHT	REPS	WEIGHT	REPS	WEIGHT	REPS

One Arm
Dumbbell Rows
on Bench
Ref: PLATE # 6

Shoulder Front
Raises
Ref: PLATE # 5

Std. Pull Ups
Ref: PLATE # 10

Shoulder Press
Ref: PLATE # 10

Narrow Grip Pull
Ups
Ref: PLATE # 11

Shoulder Lateral
Raises
Ref: PLATE # 9

Wide Pull Ups
Ref: PLATE # 11

Shoulder Press
Ref: PLATE # 10

LEGS & CORE

EXERCISE	DATE					
	WEIGHT	REPS	WEIGHT	REPS	WEIGHT	REPS
Knee Bend Lunges **Ref: PLATE # 6**						
Deep Squats **Ref: PLATE # 12**						
Std. Crunches **Ref: PLATE # 7**						
Straight Back-Leg Lunges **Ref: PLATE # 12**						
Calf Raises **Ref: PLATE # 13**						
Piano Crunches **Ref: PLATE # 13**						
Chair Pose Hold **Ref: PLATE # 14**						
Demi Squats **Ref: PLATE # 14**						
Reverse Crunches **Ref: PLATE # 7**						

CARDIO

DAY / DATE	TYPE OF EXERCISE	RESISTANCE	INCLINE / OTHER	DURATION	CALORIES BURNT

CARDIO

DAY / DATE	TYPE OF EXERCISE	RESISTANCE	INCLINE / OTHER	DURATION	CALORIES BURNT

RESTING WEEK

DAY/DATE	TYPE OF EXERCISE	Number	Notes
	Sun Salutations		
	Sun Salutations		
	Sun Salutations		
	Sun Salutations		
	Sun Salutations		
	Sun Salutations		
	Sun Salutations		
	Sun Salutations		
	Sun Salutations		
	Sun Salutations		
	Sun Salutations		
	Sun Salutations		

My Notes: *Include areas you need to improve, ease or difficulty while exercising etc. on this page ...*

Did I achieve my goals?

Which ones did I not achieve?

Why could I not achieve them?

What were my strengths?

What setbacks did I encounter?

PICTURE PLATES 1 - 14

Refer to these plates to ensure correct form & posture.

PLATE 1 – EXERCISES

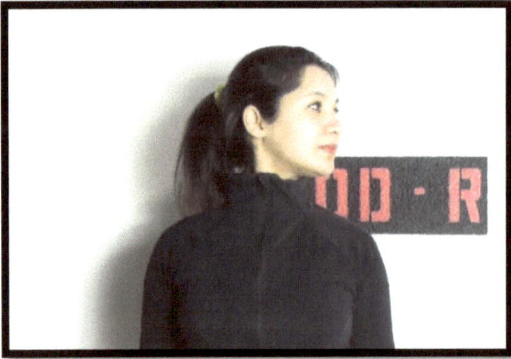

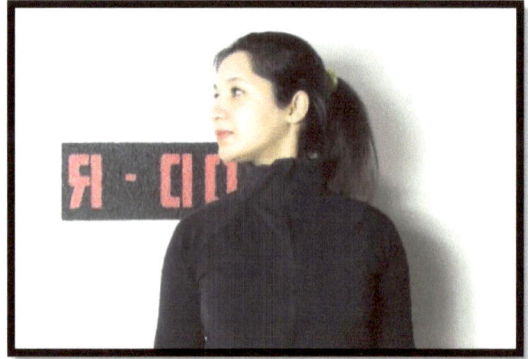

Neck Stretch: Side to Side (8 – 10 ct. each)

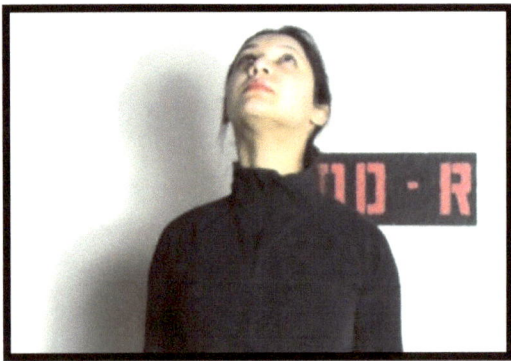

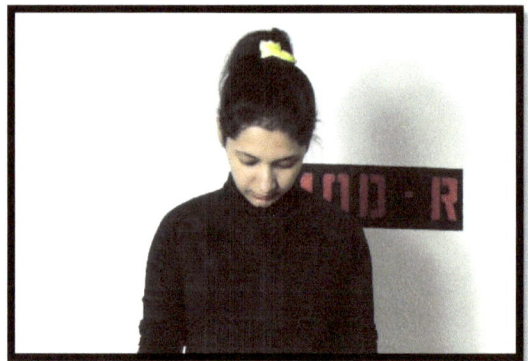

Neck Stretch: Up and Down (8 – 10 ct. each)

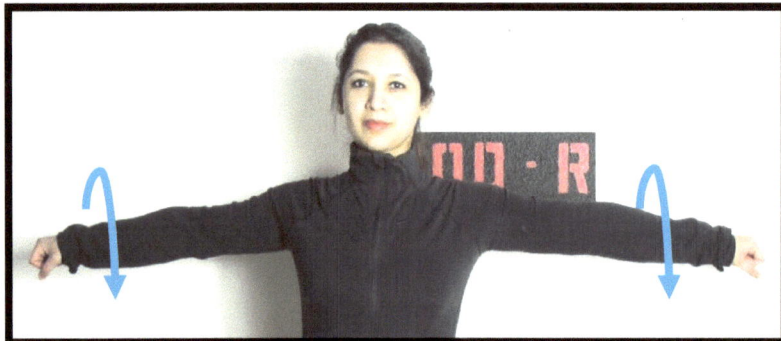

Arm Circles: Forward and Back (20 ct. each)

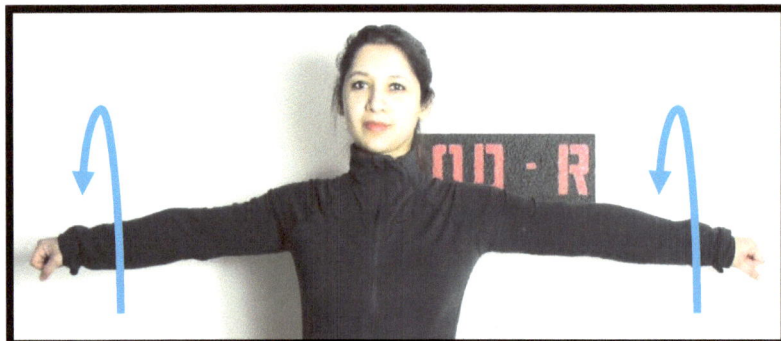

PLATE 2 – EXERCISES

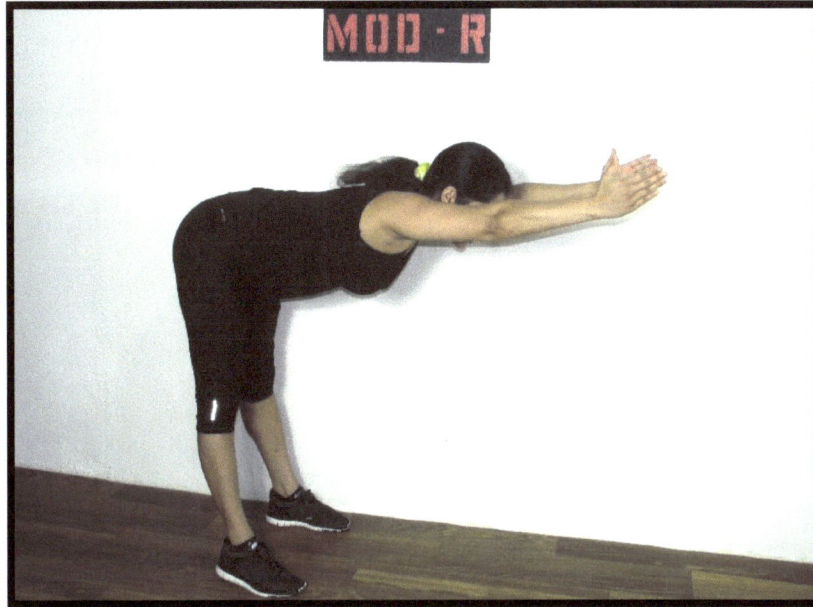

Flat Back Hamstrings Stretch (Hold: 15 – 20 sec.).
Do not bend in your knees. Back flat.

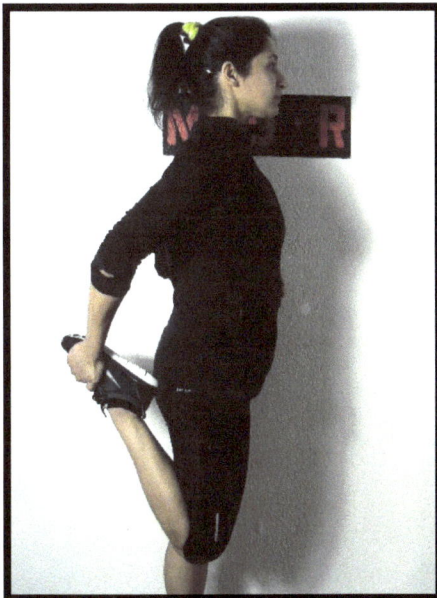

Quadriceps Stretch:
Left and Right Legs
(Hold: 20 sec. each)

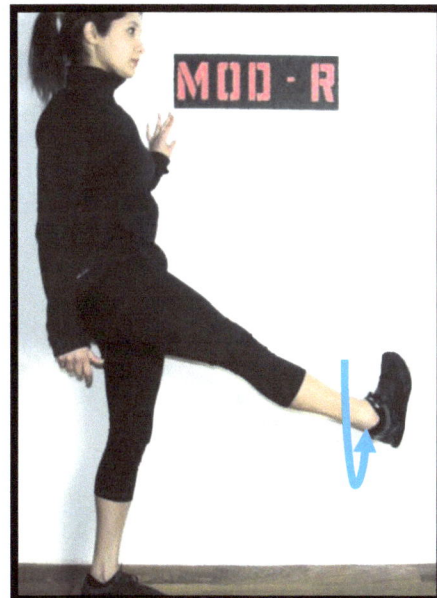

Foot Circles:
Left and Right Feet
(10 ct. each)

PLATE 3 – EXERCISES

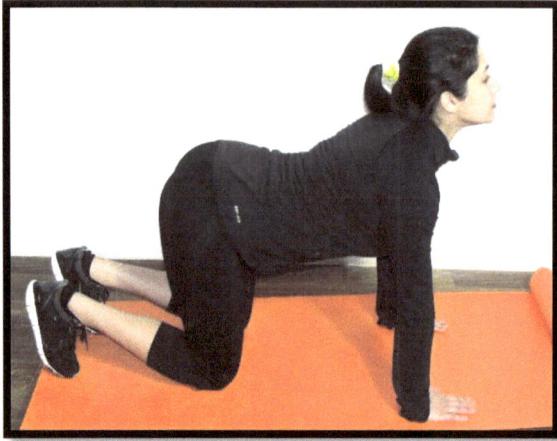

Cat Stretch:
Inhale, look up

Cat Stretch
(3 – 5 ct.)

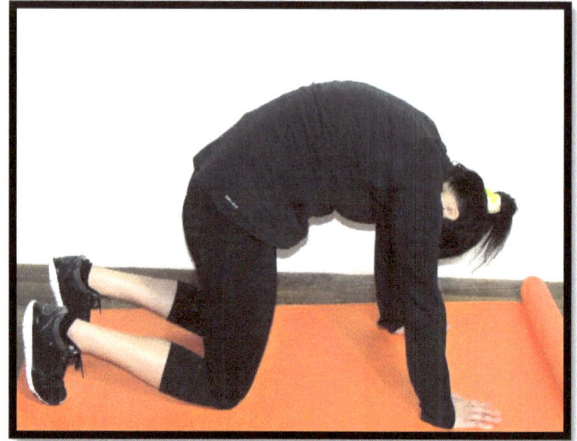

Cat Stretch:
Exhale, look down

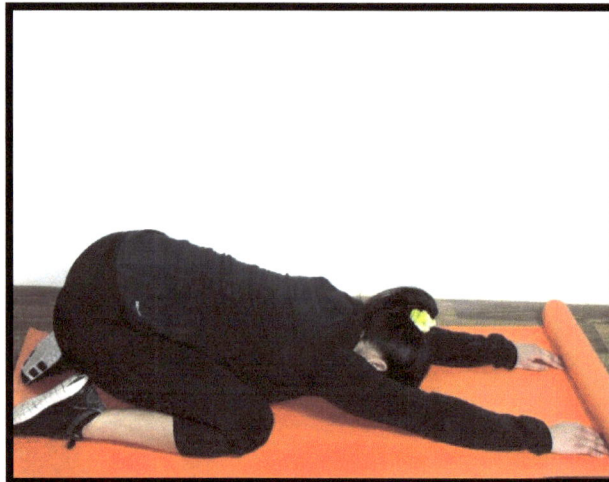

Child's Pose
(Hold: 15 – 20 sec.)

PLATE 4 – EXERCISES

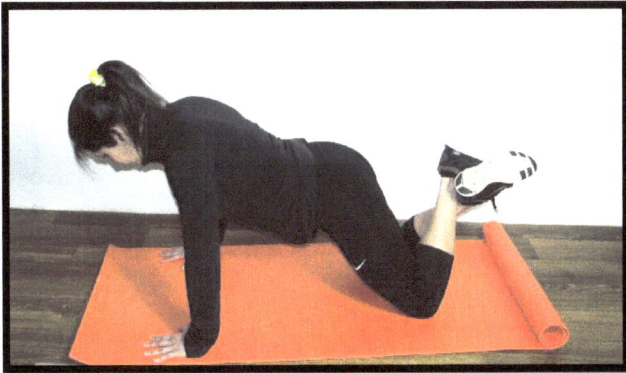

Std. Push Ups (Knees): Start

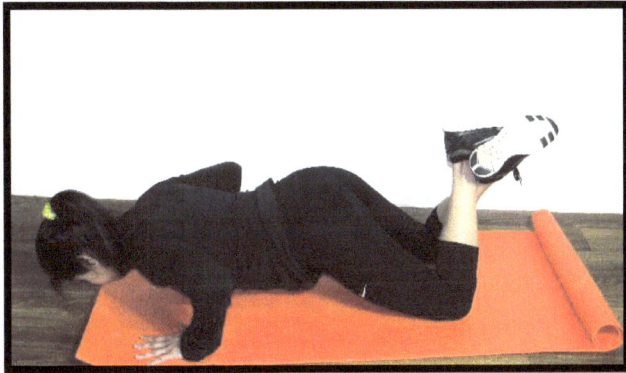

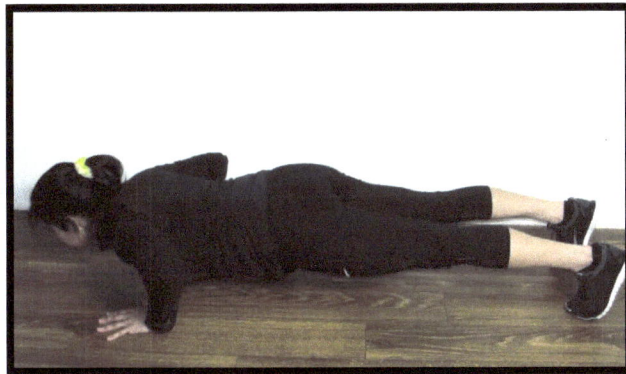

Std. Push Ups (Knees): End

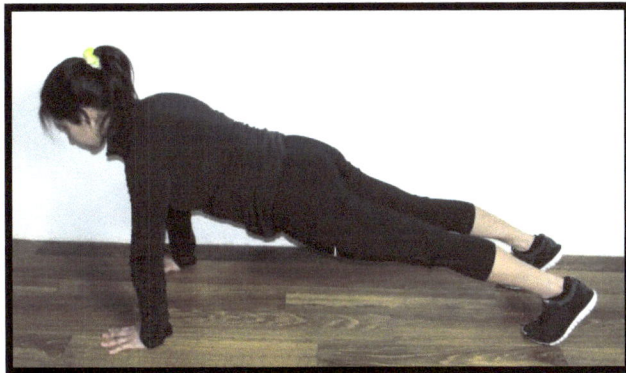

Std. Push Ups: Start

Std. Push Ups: End

Standard Push Ups:
Place hands slightly outside shoulder width.

PLATE 5 – EXERCISES

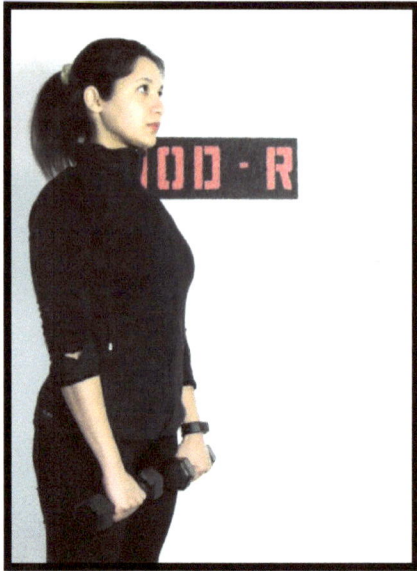

Shoulder Front Raises:
Start

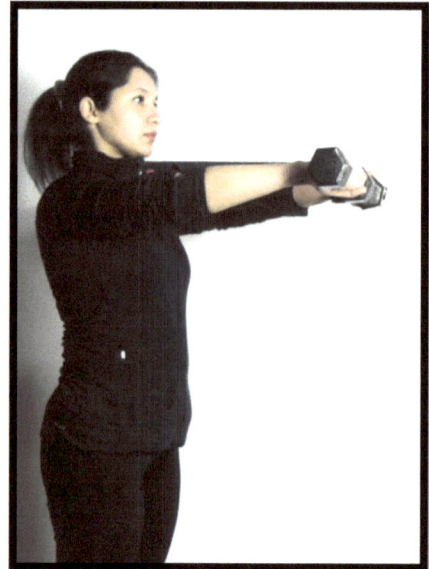

Shoulder Front Raises:
End

Shoulder Front Raises:
Elbows soft. Back straight. Raise up to shoulder level.

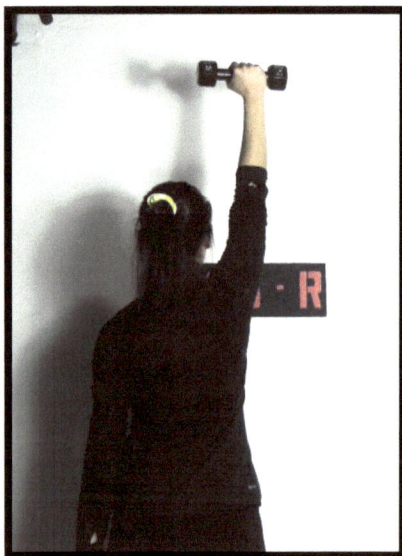

Triceps Extensions:
Start

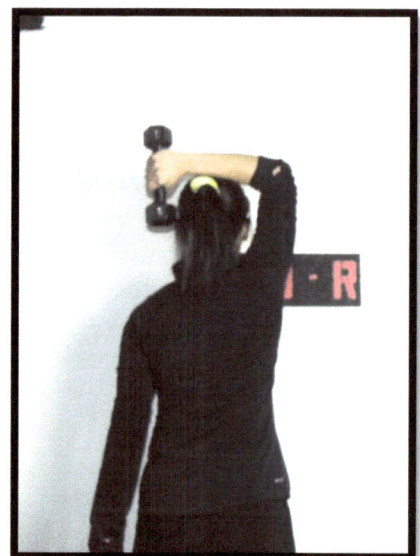

Triceps Extensions:
End

Triceps Extensions:
Perform exercise on both arms; Keep elbows soft on top. **<u>DO NOT</u>** use any weights initially. Add a very light weight once comfortable.
<u>CAUTION</u>: Avoid head injury.

PLATE 6 – EXERCISES

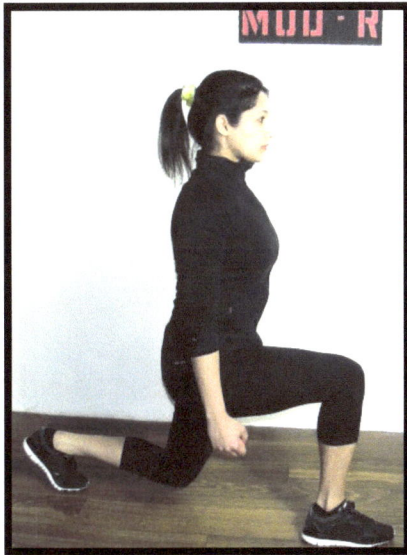

Knee-bend Lunge: Right

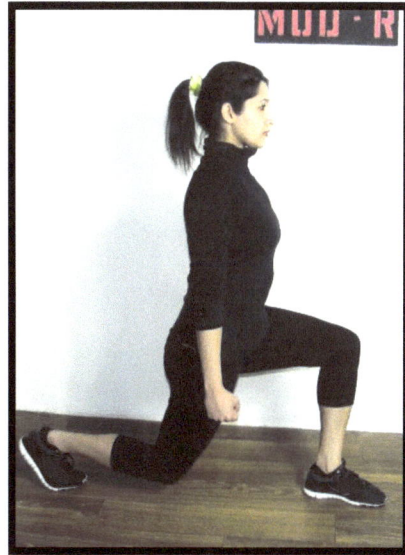

Knee-bend Lunge: Left

Lunges:
Maintain a 90° angle in front leg. Knees are in line with ankles.

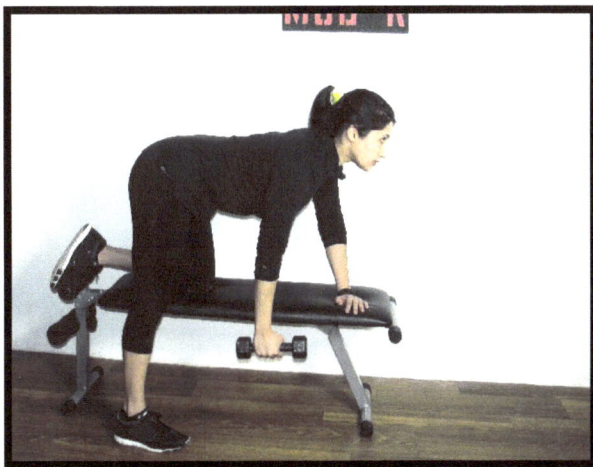

One Arm Dumbbell Rows:
Start

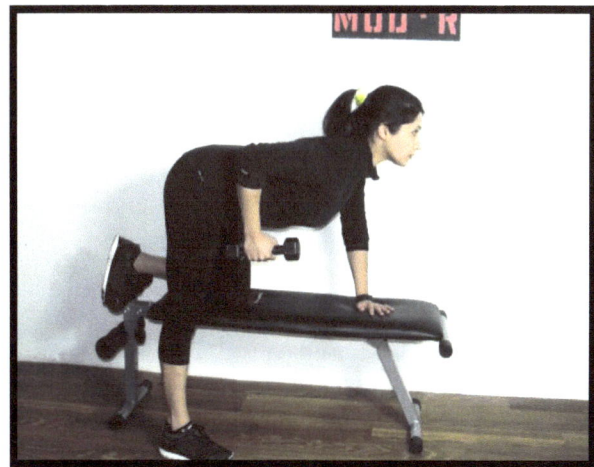

One Arm Dumbbell Rows:
End

One Arm Dumbbell Rows:
Perform Exercise for both Left and Right sides.
Back should be flat and even. Soft elbow for supporting arm.

PLATE 7 – EXERCISES

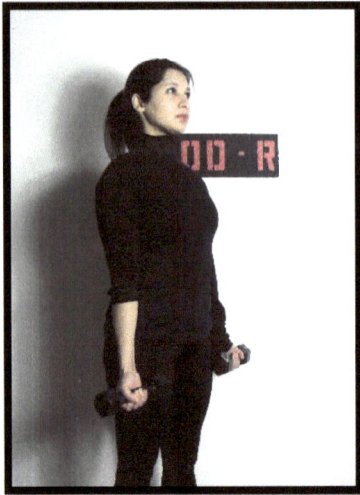

Standard Biceps Curls:
Start

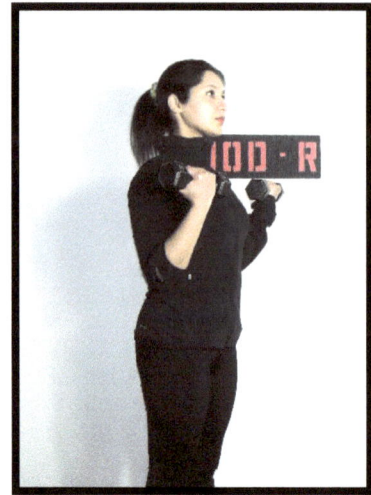

Standard Biceps Curls:
End

Std. Biceps Curls:
Hands in line with forearms. Do not drop your wrists.

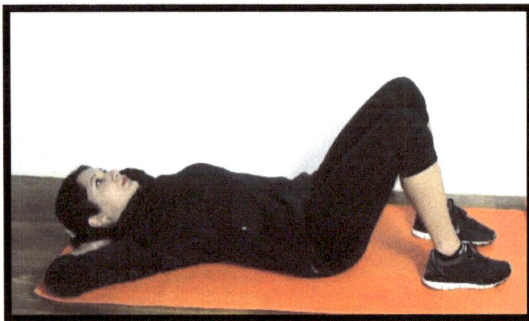

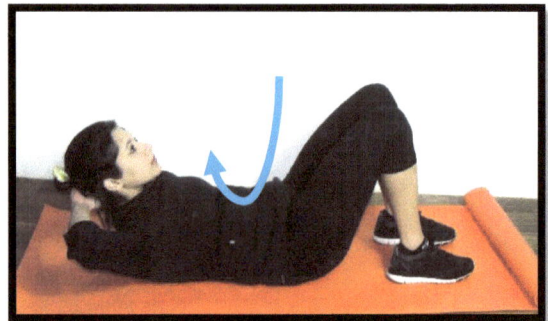

Std. Crunches:
Inhale: Going down to starting position;
Exhale: Crunching up

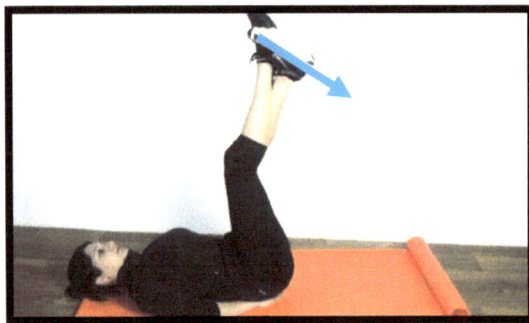

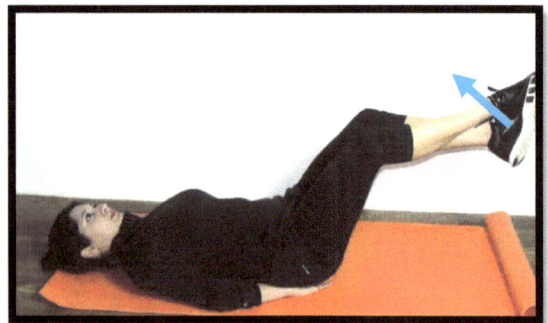

Reverse Crunches:
Inhale: Legs going down; Exhale: Legs going up

PLATE 8 – EXERCISES

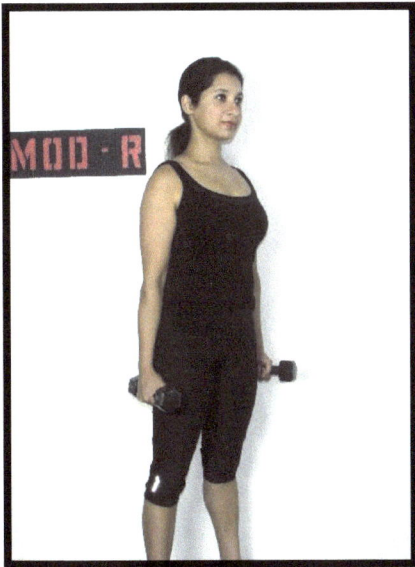

Hammer Biceps Curls:
Start

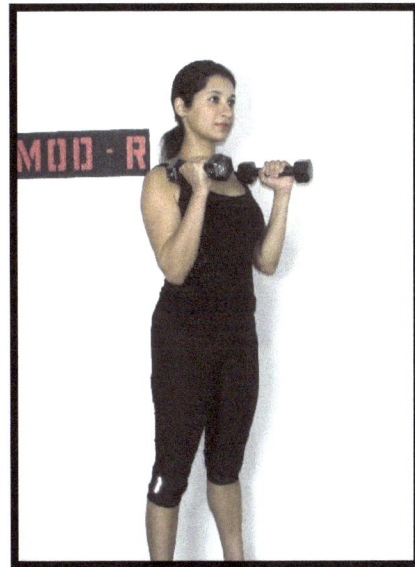

Hammer Biceps Curls:
End

Hammer Biceps Curls:
Notice the "hammer hold". Keep feet hip width apart.

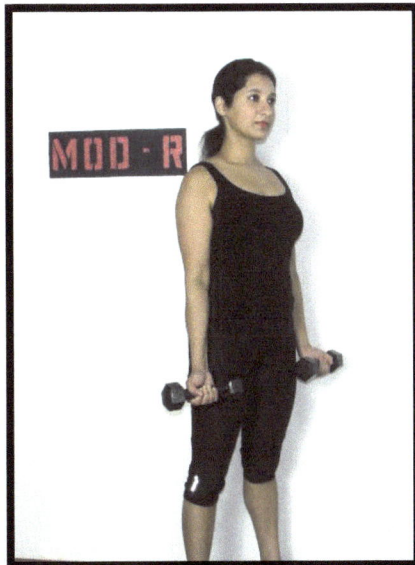

Single Arm Biceps Curls:
Start

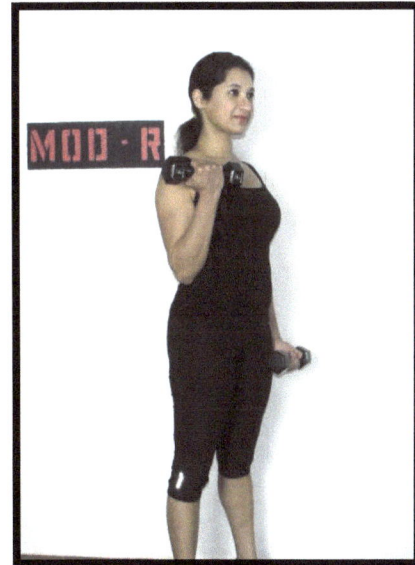

Single Arm Biceps Curls:
End

Single Arm Biceps Curls:
Perform Exercise on both arms.
Hands in line with forearms. Do not drop your wrists.

PLATE 9 – EXERCISES

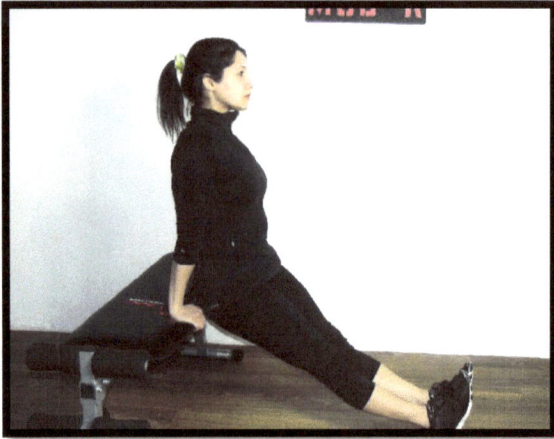

Triceps Dips: Start

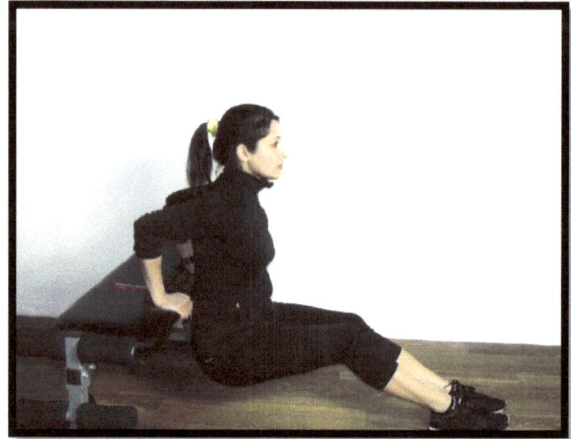

Triceps Dips : End

Triceps Dips:
Do not flare your elbows out to the side. Do not go too deep.

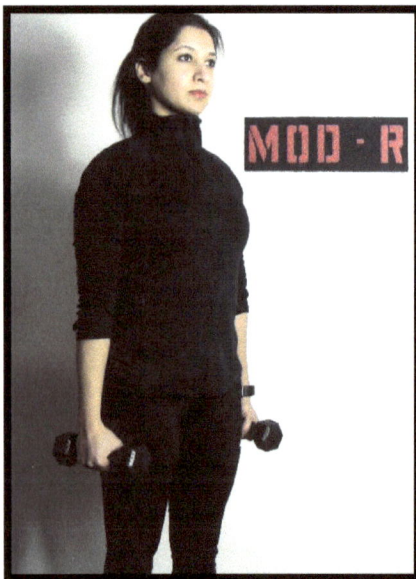

Shoulder Lateral Raises:
Start

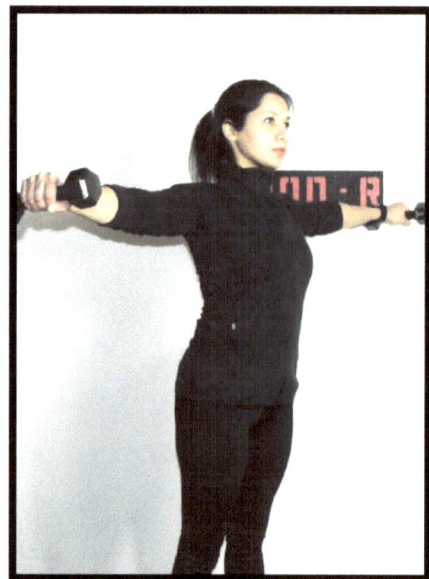

Shoulder Lateral Raises:
End

Shoulder Lateral Raises:
Back straight. Do not go above shoulder level.

PLATE 10 – EXERCISES

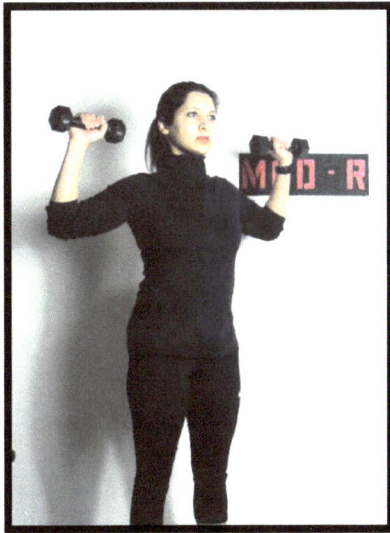

Shoulder Press: Start

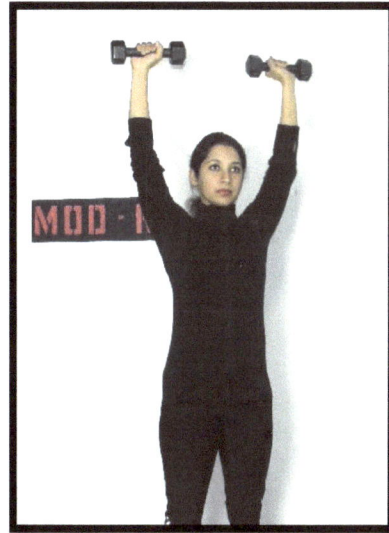

Shoulder Press: End

Shoulder Press:
Start with the dumbbells at ear level. Keep a straight back.
Keep soft elbows at the top. Use lower weights.

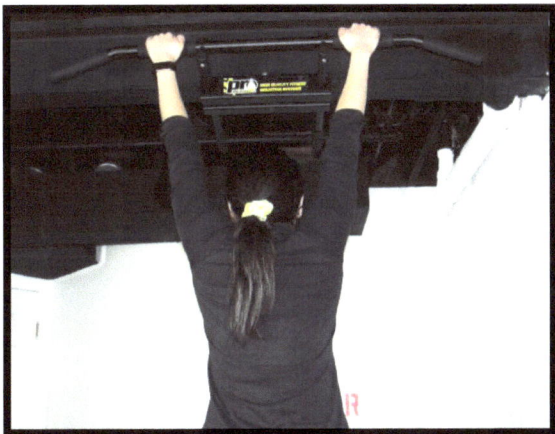

Std. Pull Ups: Start

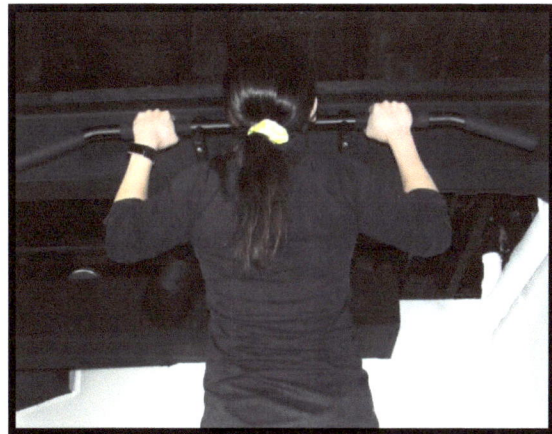

Std. Pull Ups: End

Standard Pull Ups:
Arms slightly outside shoulder width.
Use assists such as bands or a simple chair to support your legs.

PLATE 11 – EXERCISES

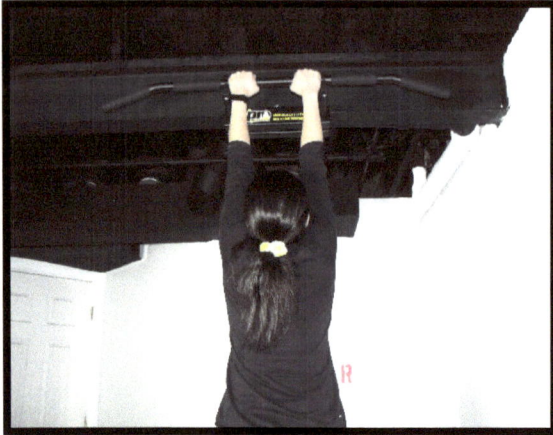

Narrow Grip Pull Ups: Start

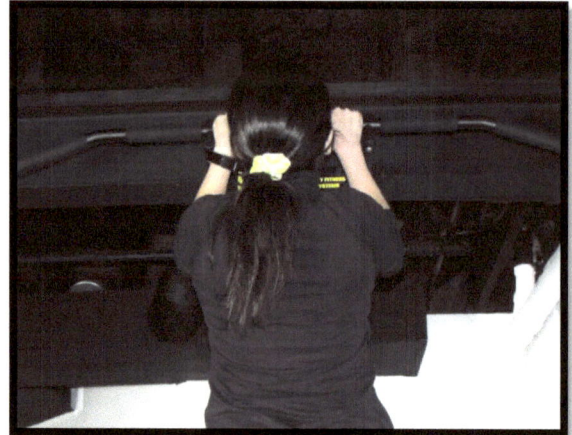

Narrow Grip Pull Ups: End

Narrow Grip Pull Ups:
Arms in line with shoulders.
Use assists such as bands or a simple chair to support your legs.

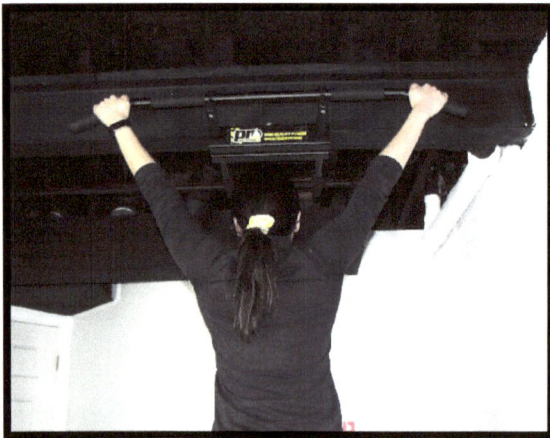

Wide Pull Ups: Start

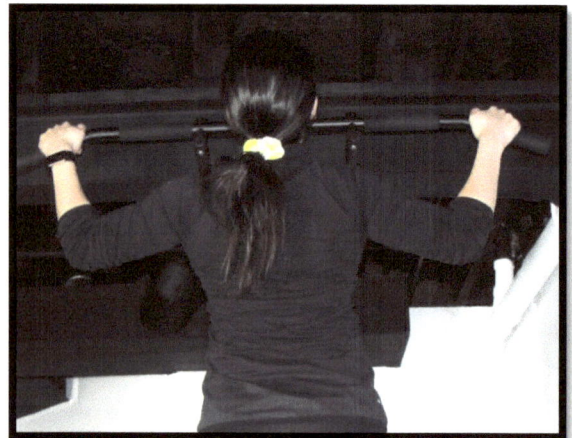

Wide Pull Ups: End

Wide Pull Ups:
Arms wide outside shoulder width.
Use assists such as bands or a simple chair to support your legs.

PLATE 12 – EXERCISES

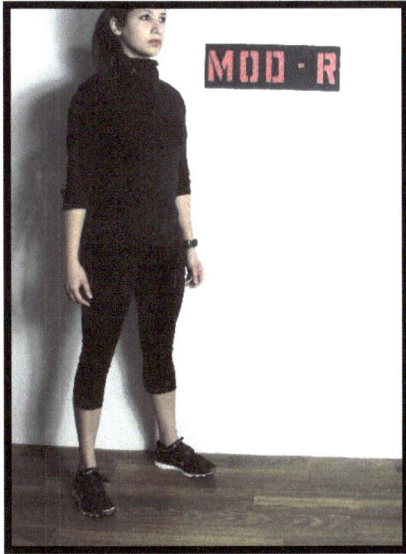

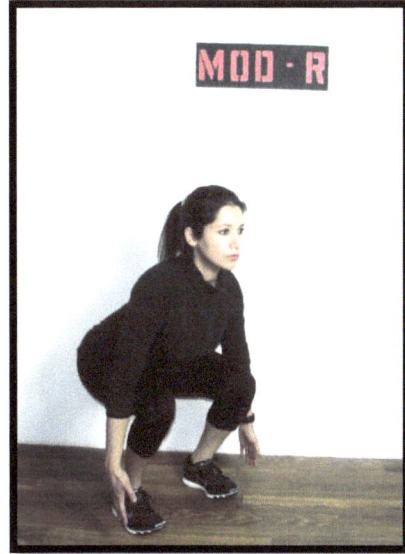

Deep Squats: Start   Deep Squats: End

Deep Squats:
Maintain body weight on heels. Keep toes raised.
Do not go deep if it is uncomfortable.

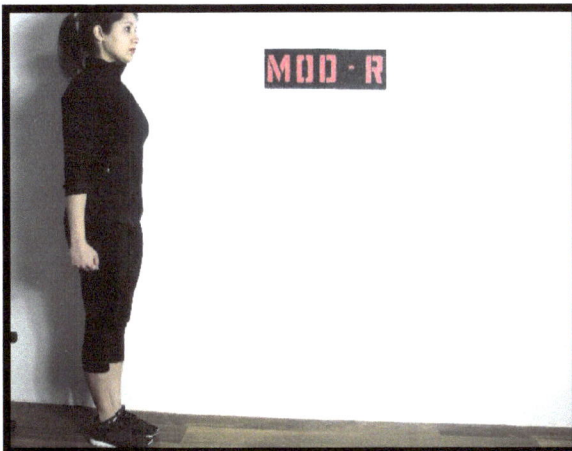

Straight Back-Leg Lunges: Start   Straight Back-Leg Lunges: End

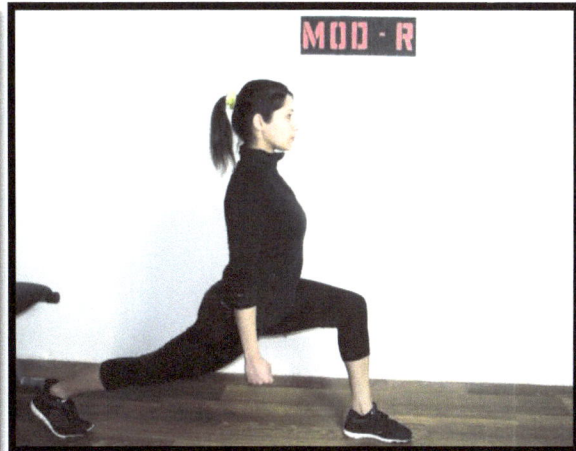

Straight Back-Leg Lunges:
Perform exercise on both legs.
Back leg is straight. Front leg knee at 90° angle.

PLATE 13 – EXERCISES

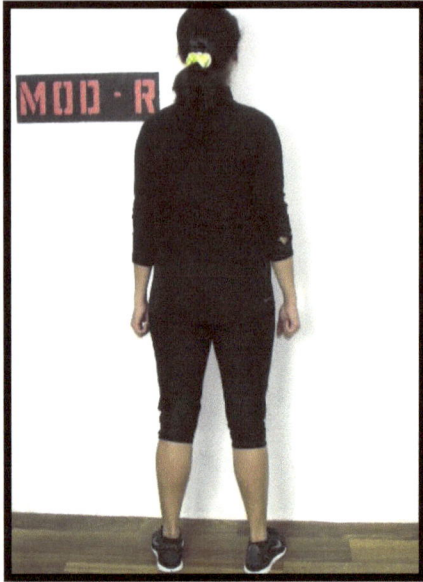

Calf Raises: Start

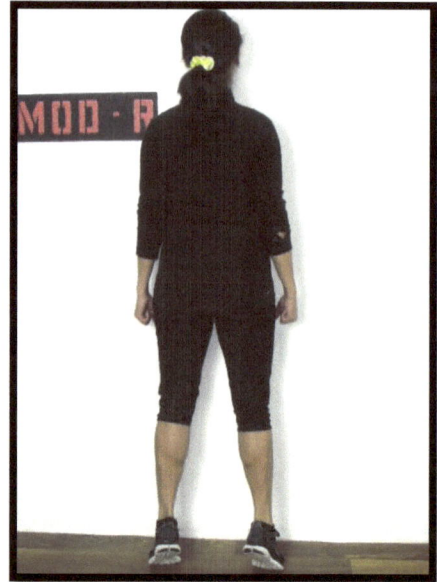

Calf Raises: End

Calf Raises:
Feet hip width apart. Toes pointing slightly outwards. Raise your heels off the ground and back.

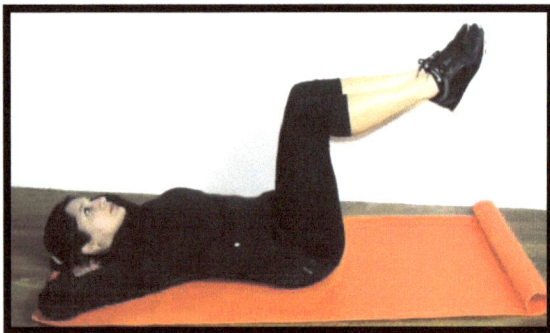

Piano Crunches: Start

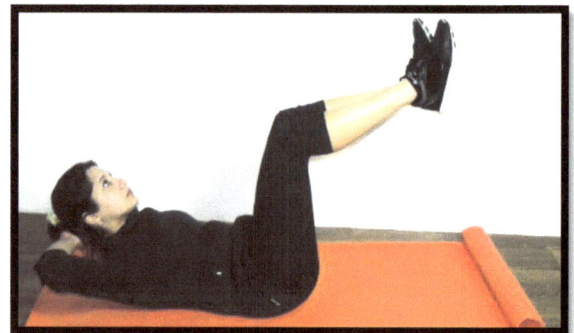

Piano Crunches: End

Piano Crunches:
Exhale as you crunch up.
Inhale as you go back to starting position.

PLATE 14 – EXERCISES

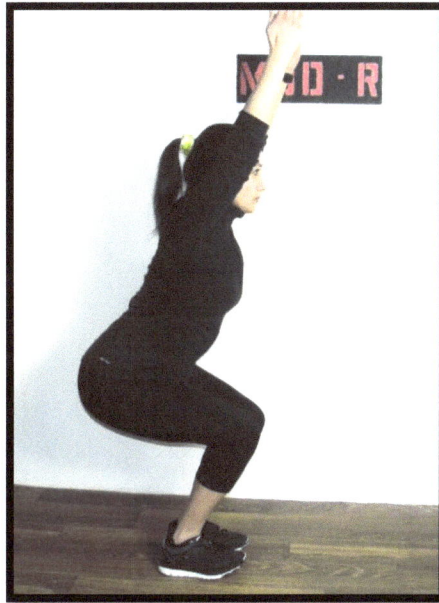

Chair Pose:
Hold and record duration as you progress.
Body weight on heels. Back straight.

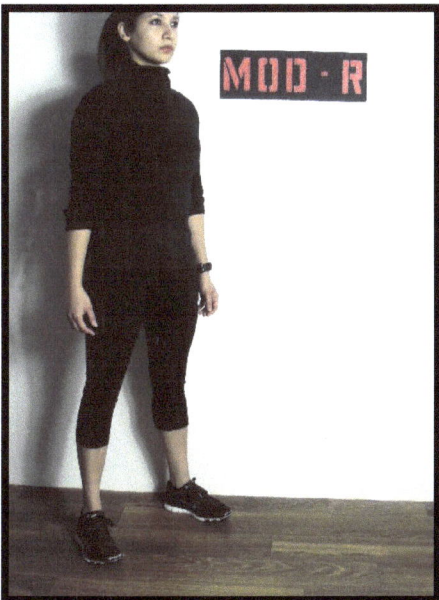

Demi Squats: Start

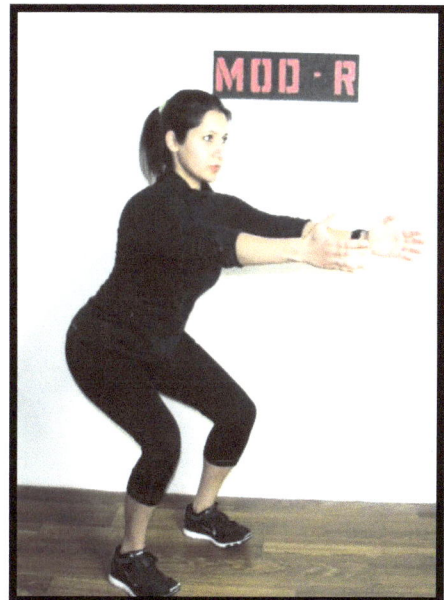

Demi Squats: End

Demi Squats:
Body weight on heels.

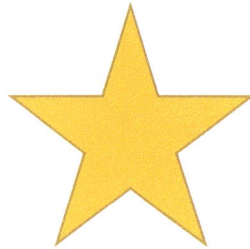

CONGRATULATIONS!

You have completed the **Basic Wellness Program Levels 1 and 2!** You are now ready to take further steps to enhanced fitness!

My New Plans...

Follow us on –

Facebook:
@modRwellness

Instagram:
@modrwellness
#richamodak
#modRwellness
#horseridingdietitian

YouTube:
Richa Modak

www.ingramcontent.com/pod-product-compliance
Lightning Source LLC
Chambersburg PA
CBHW060804270326
41927CB00002B/42